Cambridge **Discovery Education**™

▶ **INTERACTIVE READERS**

Series editor: Bob Hastings

SO CUTE!

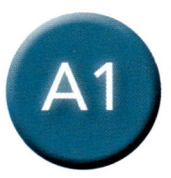

A1

Kenna Bourke

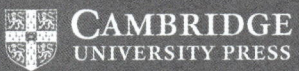

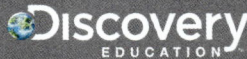

CAMBRIDGE
UNIVERSITY PRESS

University Printing House, Cambridge CB2 8BS, United Kingdom

One Liberty Plaza, 20th Floor, New York, NY 10006, USA

477 Williamstown Road, Port Melbourne, VIC 3207, Australia

4843/24, 2nd Floor, Ansari Road, Daryaganj, Delhi – 110002, India

79 Anson Road, #06–04/06, Singapore 079906

Cambridge University Press is part of the University of Cambridge.

It furthers the University's mission by disseminating knowledge in the pursuit of
education, learning and research at the highest international levels of excellence.

www.cambridge.org
Information on this title: www.cambridge.org/9781107646490

© Cambridge University Press 2014

This publication is in copyright. Subject to statutory exception
and to the provisions of relevant collective licensing agreements,
no reproduction of any part may take place without the written
permission of Cambridge University Press.

First published 2014
20 19 18 17 16 15 14 13 12 11 10 9 8 7

Printed in Dubai by Oriental Press

A catalogue record for this publication is available from the British Library.

Library of Congress Cataloguing in Publication data
Bourke, Kenna.
 So cute! / Kenna Bourke.
    pages cm. -- (Cambridge discovery interactive readers)
 ISBN 978-1-107-64649-0 (pbk. : alk. paper)
1. Beauty, Personal--Juvenile literature. 2. English language--Textbooks for foreign speakers.
3. Readers (Elementary) I. Title.

GT499.B68 2013
391.6--dc23

2013025112

ISBN 978-1-107-64649-0

Additional resources for this publication at www.cambridge.org

Cambridge University Press has no responsibility for the persistence or accuracy
of URLs for external or third-party internet websites referred to in this publication,
and does not guarantee that any content on such websites is, or will remain,
accurate or appropriate.

Layout services, art direction, book design, and photo research: Q2ABillSMITH GROUP
Editorial services: Hyphen S.A.
Audio production: CityVox, New York
Video production: Q2ABillSMITH GROUP

Contents

Before You Read: Get Ready! 4

CHAPTER 1
That's So Cute! 6

CHAPTER 2
Babies, Adults, and Older Adults 8

CHAPTER 3
Kittens and Puppies 12

CHAPTER 4
A World of Cute 16

CHAPTER 5
What Do You Think? 20

After You Read 22

Answer Key 24

Glossary

Before You Read:
Get Ready!

Cute means "easy to like." We see cute things all the time, but what is cute, really? Why are some things cute and others aren't?

Words to Know

Look at the pictures. Then complete the sentences below with the correct words.

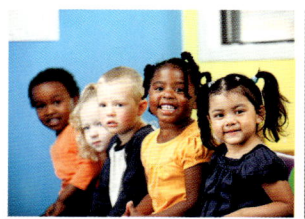
kids

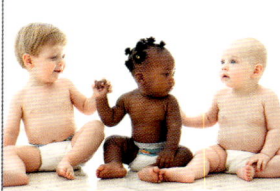
human babies

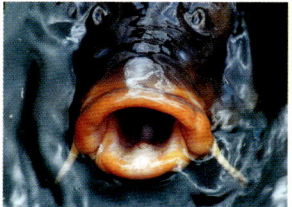
ugly

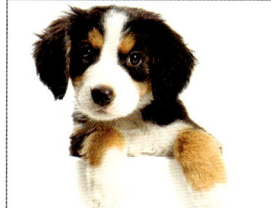
puppy

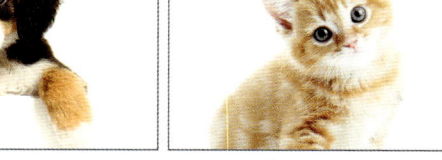
kitten

1 Some fish are very _____, but others are beautiful.

2 _____ can't walk or talk when they're born.

3 A _____ is a baby dog.

4 Another word for children is _____.

5 A _____ is a baby cat.

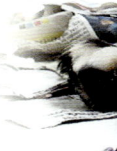

Words to Know

Read the paragraph. Then complete the sentences below with the correct highlighted words.

People and most animals are helpless when they are babies. They can't do anything. This means the parents – or other older people – have to do everything for them. We often say that babies are innocent – they don't know about bad things. They don't know much about life, and they can easily make mistakes. Something in our brains tells us we must help them and protect them.

1. We use our _____ to think.

2. The puppy is one day old. It's _____ and needs its mother.

3. Adults know there are bad things in the world. They aren't _____ .

4. A hat can _____ your head from cold weather and rain.

5. There are _____ in your e-mail. Check your writing.

6. John is four years old. Meg is two. John is _____ than Meg.

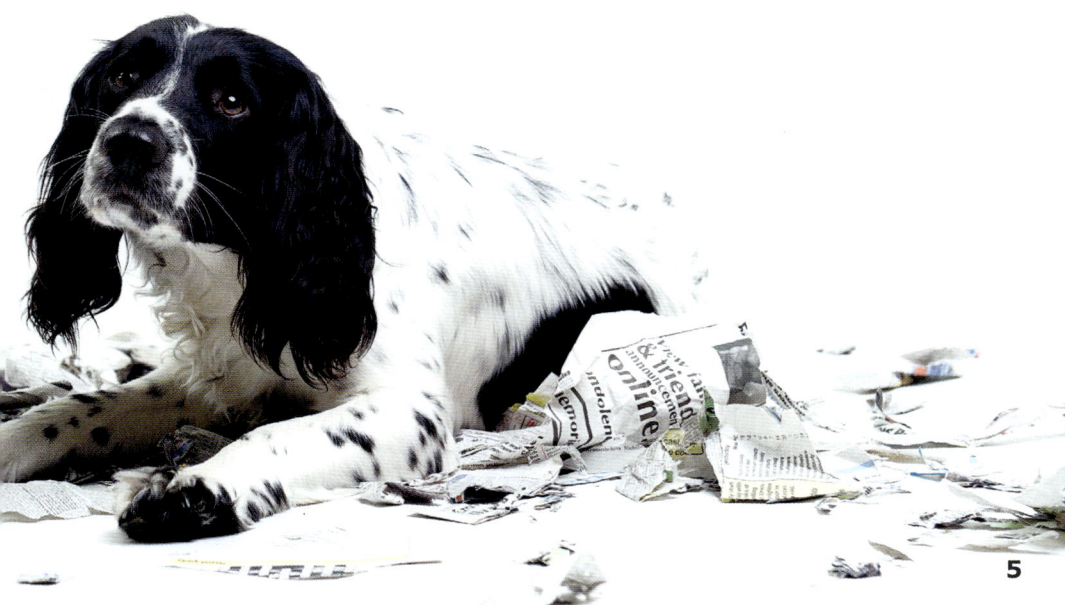

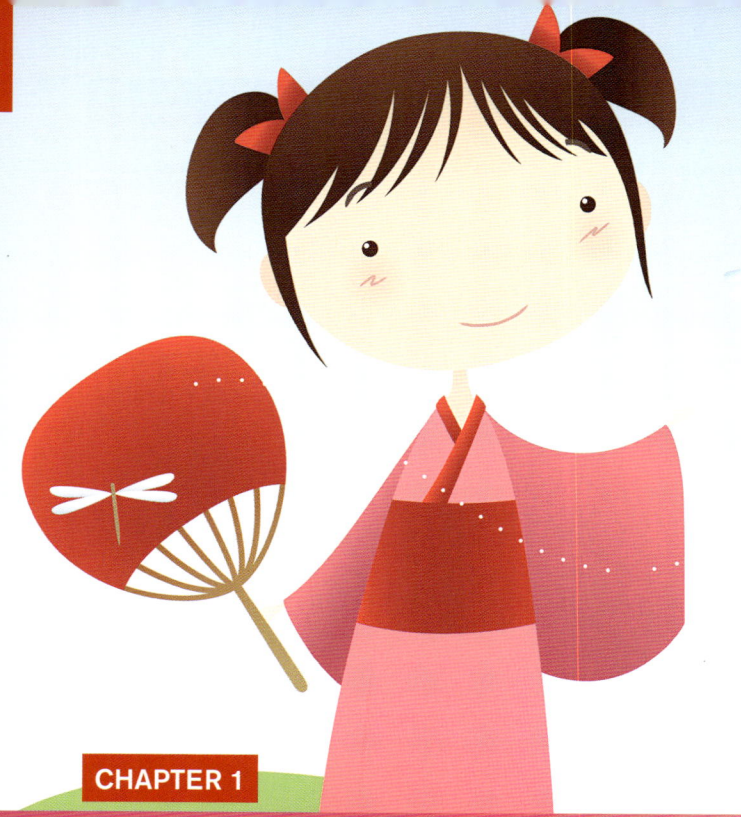

CHAPTER 1

That's So Cute!

**"OH! THAT'S SO CUTE!"
HOW OFTEN DO YOU HEAR THESE WORDS?**

Do we all think the same things are cute? Yes, mostly we do.

Babies, **even** the ugly ones, are cute. So are adults with round, childlike faces – big eyes, small chins and noses, and big foreheads. Small animals are cute. Babies learning to walk are cute. The question is *why*?

Well, it's because being cute helps you to **survive**. Something in our brains tells us what's cute, and what's not cute. We want to help cute people and animals.

Is it only living things that are cute? No! Pictures can be cute, too. Here's how to draw a picture of a cute person:

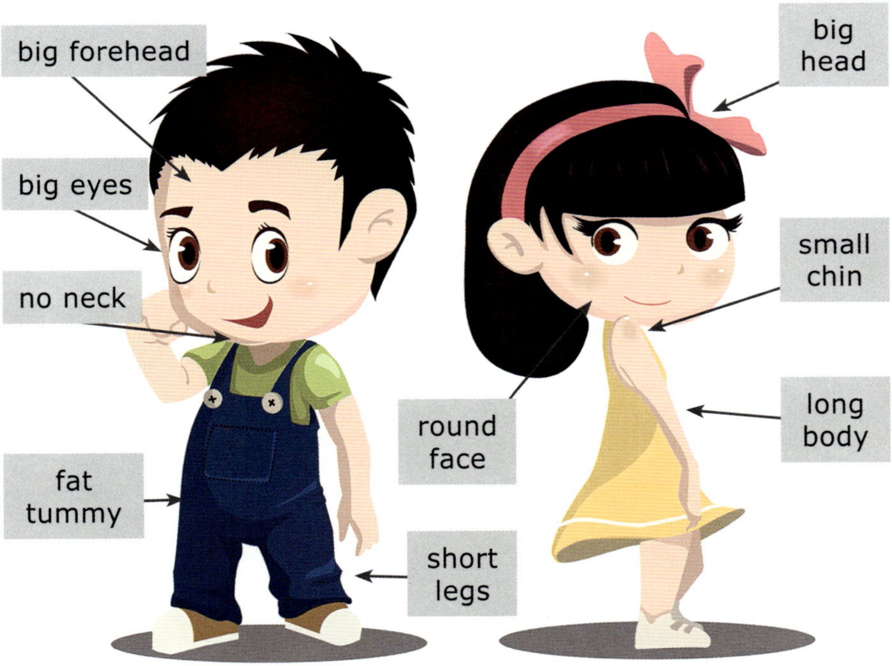

big forehead

big eyes

no neck

fat tummy

big head

small chin

long body

round face

short legs

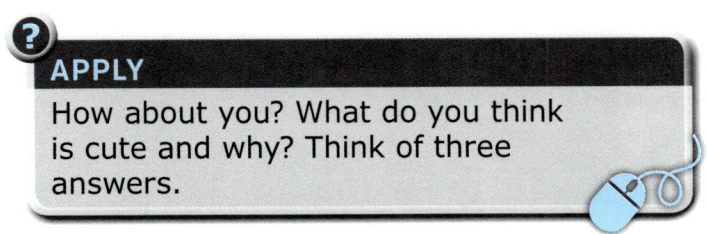

?

APPLY

How about you? What do you think is cute and why? Think of three answers.

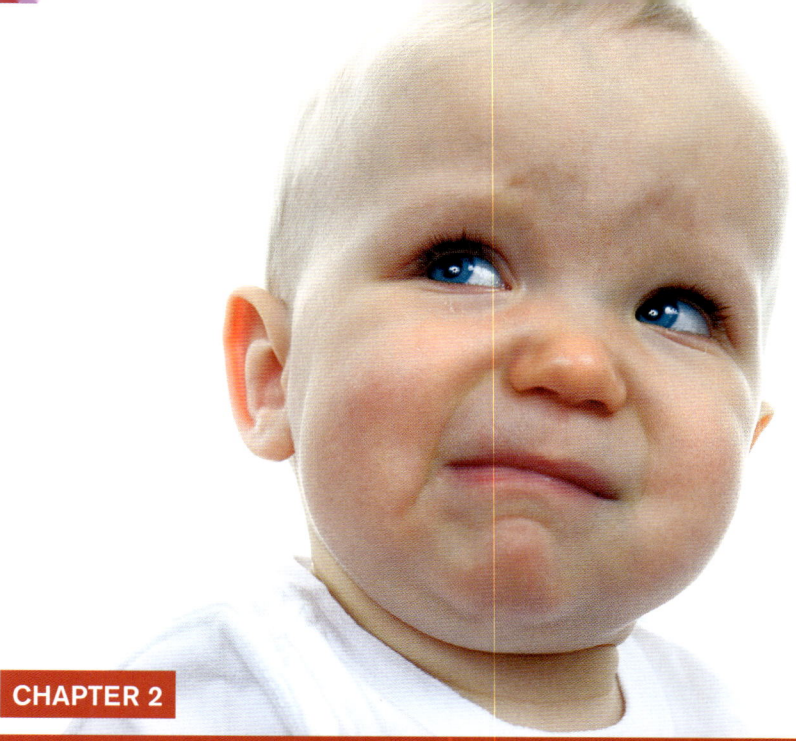

CHAPTER 2

Babies, Adults, and Older Adults

WHAT MAKES PEOPLE CUTE?

It's funny, isn't it? Babies can't do anything but eat, cry, and stop us from sleeping at night. But we think they're very cute, and we want to do everything for them!

OK, so babies **look** cute with their fat legs and arms and their big round eyes. But it's not only how they look that makes them cute. It's also the things they do.

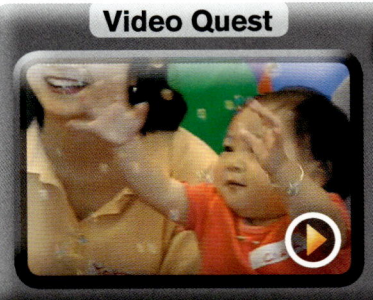

Babies and Bubbles

Watch the video about babies playing. Why do parents take their children to these places?

When babies learn to speak and walk, we find them cute. This is partly because they make mistakes. They say the wrong word or say a word in a funny way. They **fall** down. And it's the same with animals. Think of a giraffe learning to walk – lots and lots of mistakes!

But mistakes aren't always cute. Think about it. You ask a friend to dinner. He gets food on his face and orange juice on your kitchen table. You're not happy. You think your friend is disgusting.[1] But a baby does the same thing, and you think it's cute.

Babies' mistakes are cute because they are young and helpless. We humans know our babies can't survive without our help. And animals know that their babies need help to survive, too.

[1] **disgusting:** very ugly, not nice

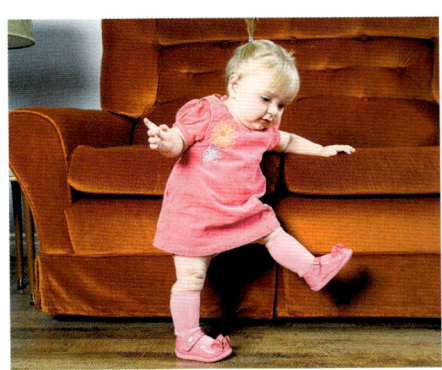

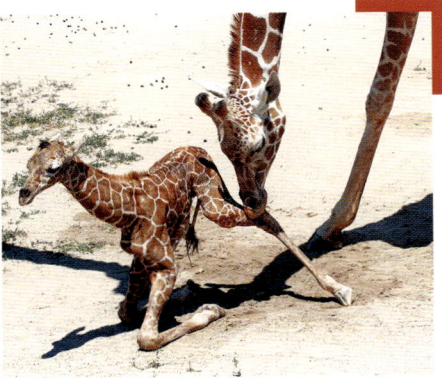

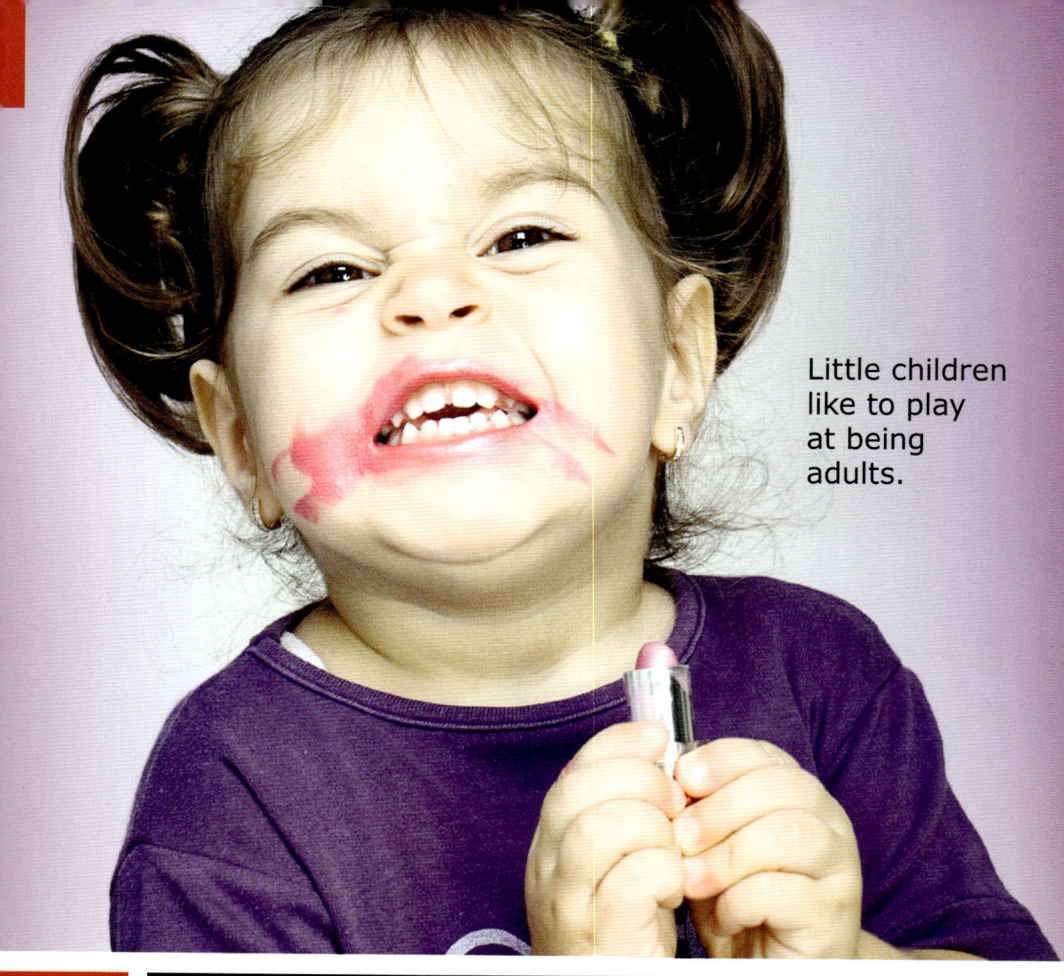

Little children like to play at being adults.

Like all living things, babies grow up – they get bigger! Do they stop being cute? Maybe a little. But kids, adults, and much older adults can still be cute.

Small children often play at being adults – they dress up in adults' clothes or put on makeup or do adult things, like "being a doctor" or "teaching school."

Parents can be cute, too. When we see the love between a parent and child, our brains tell us, that's cute!

And then there are cute old people. What makes them cute? Often, it's their **behavior**. Older people sometimes do funny things. They **behave** like young people. They show that they're in love, they start new sports, or they like to use modern[2] things like computers or smartphones.

Older people are also cute because they are a little like babies. They can be innocent, and they often need more help than younger people. Again, something in our brains tells us to protect them.

[2]**modern:** new; from today

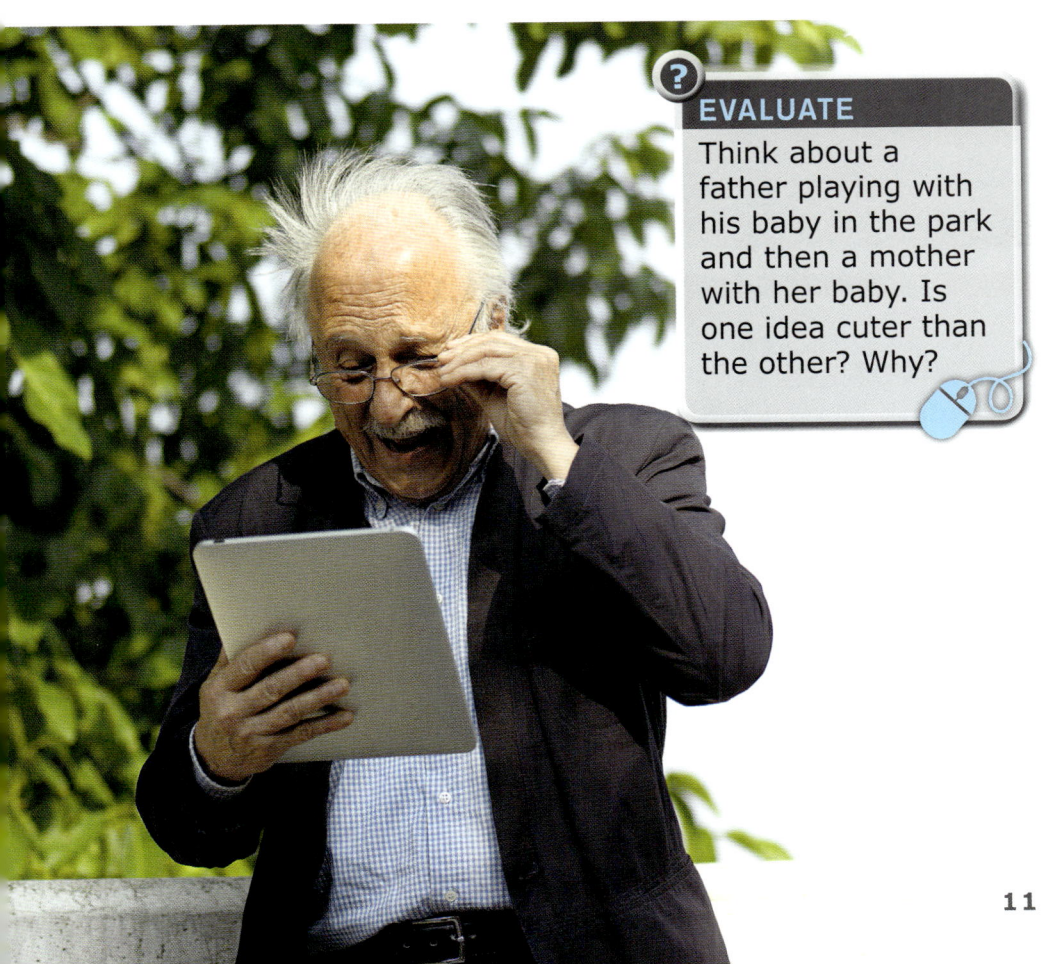

?

EVALUATE

Think about a father playing with his baby in the park and then a mother with her baby. Is one idea cuter than the other? Why?

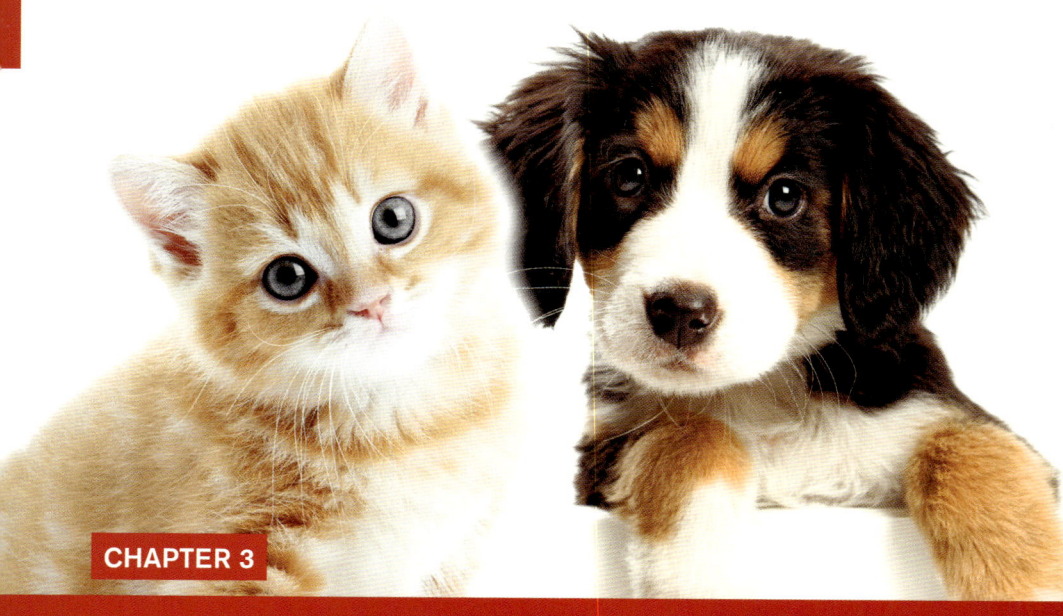

CHAPTER 3

Kittens and Puppies

WHICH IS CUTER – A KITTEN OR A PUPPY?

There are "cat people" and "dog people," but usually everybody thinks baby cats and baby dogs are very, very cute.

When animals are **newborn**, they're small and helpless. But only a few days later, they're walking and looking at the world around them. They make us **laugh** because of the funny things they do.

When we think about kids, we often think about kids playing with toys. Puppies and kittens play, too. When they play, they're having fun, but they're also learning. They're learning how to be good cats and dogs.

Sometimes puppies and kittens play with things that we don't want them to play with. For example, your puppy eats your homework or your new shoes, and that's a bad thing! Do you get angry?[3] Yes! But not for long.

[3]**angry:** the way you feel when someone does something bad to you

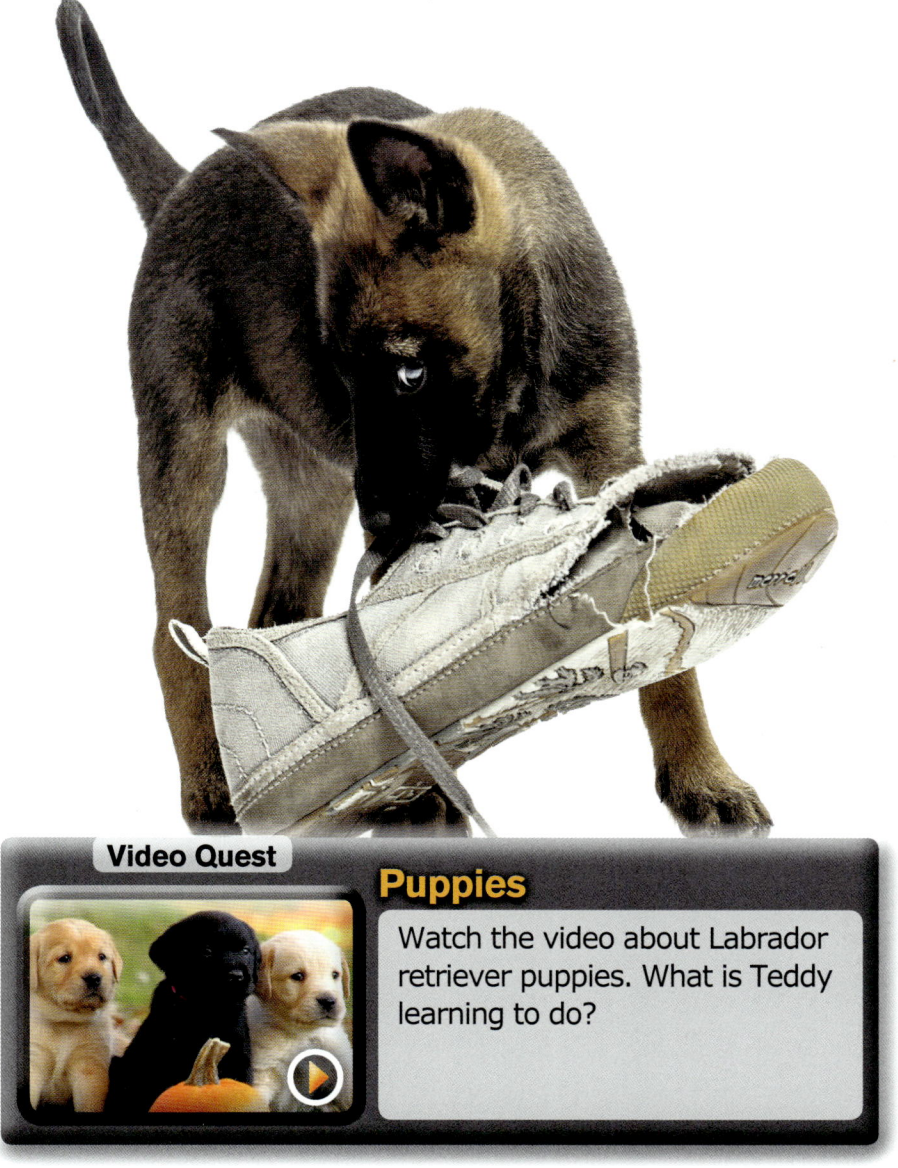

Video Quest

Puppies

Watch the video about Labrador retriever puppies. What is Teddy learning to do?

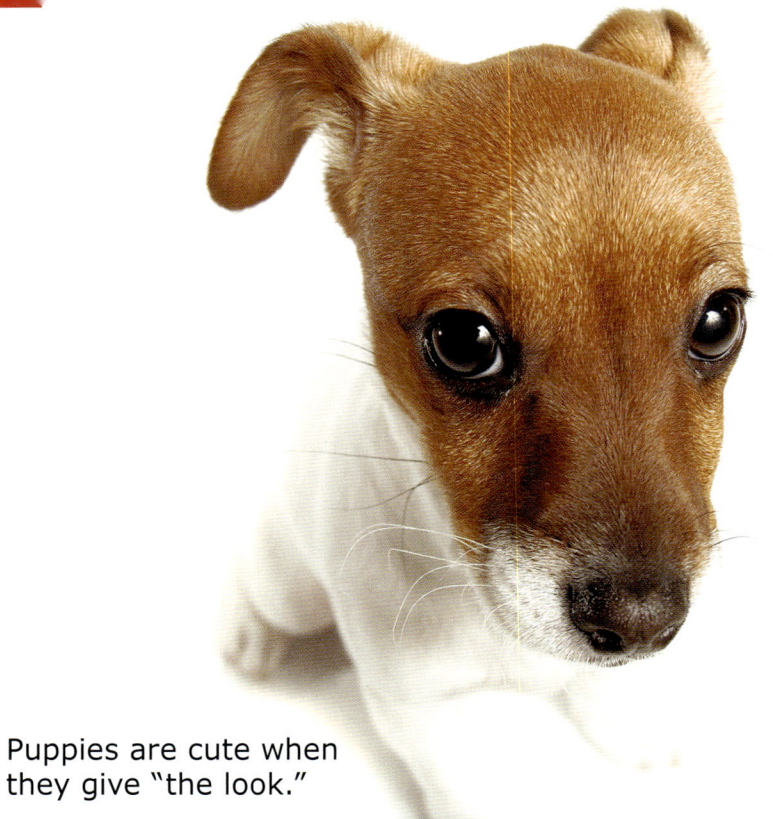

Puppies are cute when
they give "the look."

Kittens and puppies get things wrong. Like people, they make mistakes. For example, they learn to jump and run, but they fall down easily and walk into things. One minute, they're playing; the next minute they're sleeping.

Their behavior makes us say, "Aww!" But why? Maybe because we like it when animals behave like we do. And sometimes, like little children, animals behave badly. A *very bad puppy*, one who doesn't behave well, is really cute!

And of course, don't forget, THE LOOK!

Puppies and kittens can melt our hearts[4] when they look at us with their big eyes. It almost looks like they have human feelings!

Animals like cats and dogs are our friends. We feel they can understand us. They almost talk with their eyes. This is why we train, or teach, cats and dogs to be "helper animals."

Helper animals help sad or sick people feel better. Some dogs help blind people to see or deaf people to hear. Other dogs use their noses to tell doctors when people are sick!

....

[4]**melt our hearts:** make us feel like crying because of love

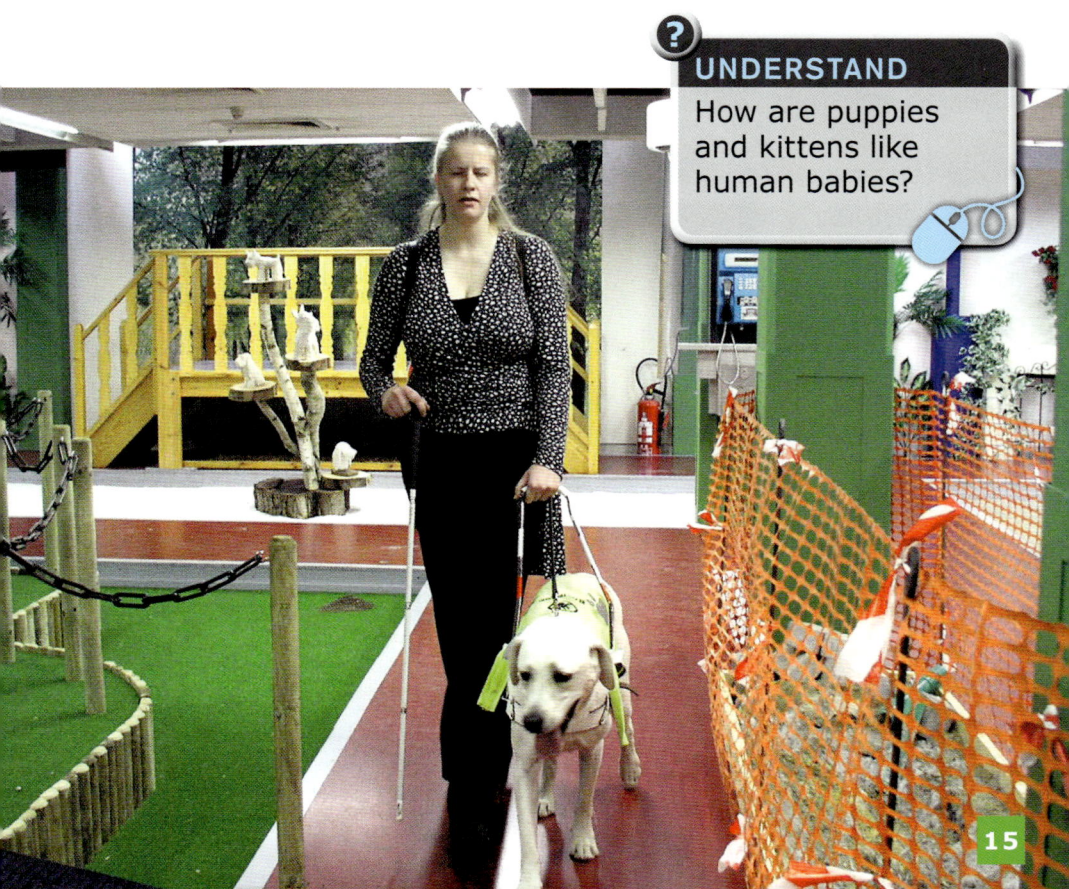

? UNDERSTAND

How are puppies and kittens like human babies?

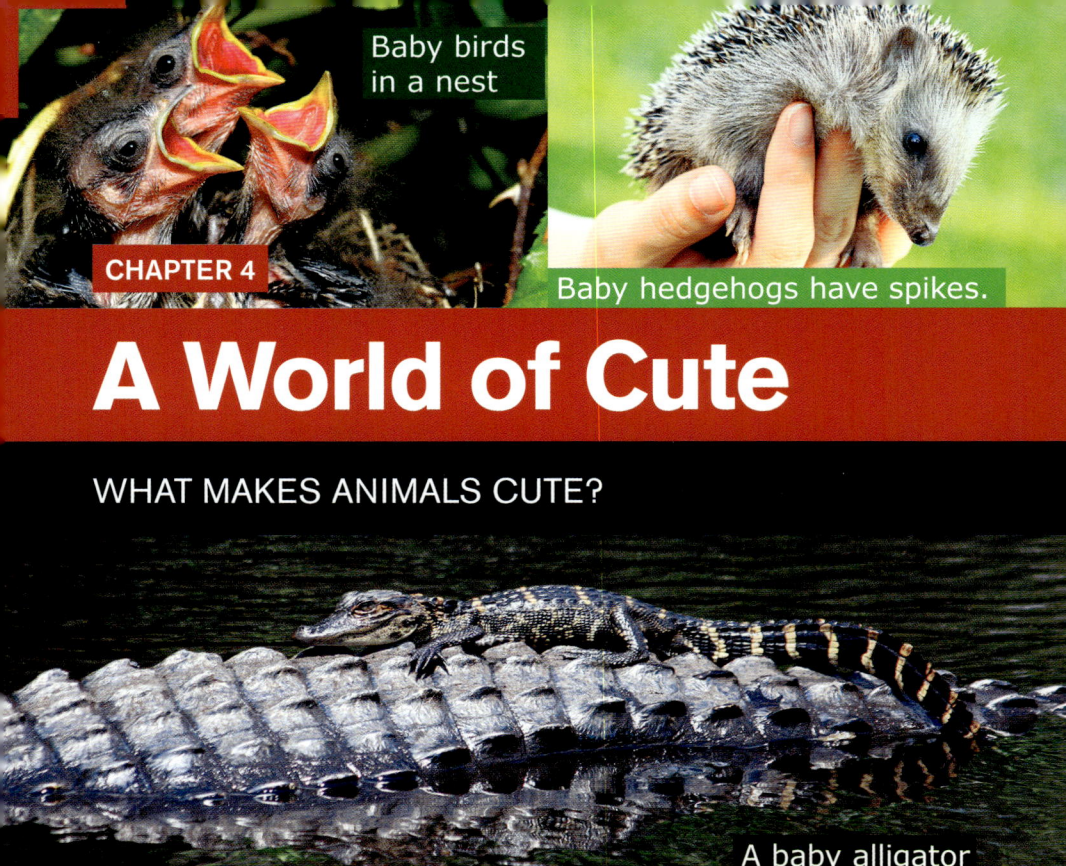

Baby birds in a nest

CHAPTER 4

Baby hedgehogs have spikes.

A World of Cute

WHAT MAKES ANIMALS CUTE?

A baby alligator

Is it just furry[5] animals that are cute? No!

Think of baby birds. Every spring,[6] there are little birds high up in trees. They sit in their nests waiting for their parents to give them food. They're cute.

Things with spikes aren't usually cute, but how about baby hedgehogs? Are they cute?

And think about **dangerous** animals like alligators with their big teeth. They aren't cute. Or are they?

[5]**furry:** with soft hair

[6]**spring:** the time of year before summer

When people really don't like each other, we say, "They fight like cats and dogs." Usually, cats don't like dogs, and dogs don't like cats. Dogs chase cats. And cats swat at dogs. Everyone knows that!

But it's not always true. Animals sometimes live together in the same house, or on the same farm. And different **species** don't always fight. They can learn to play together, sleep together, and even share the same food. Sometimes different species can be friends. And that's really cute.

Cats swat at dogs.

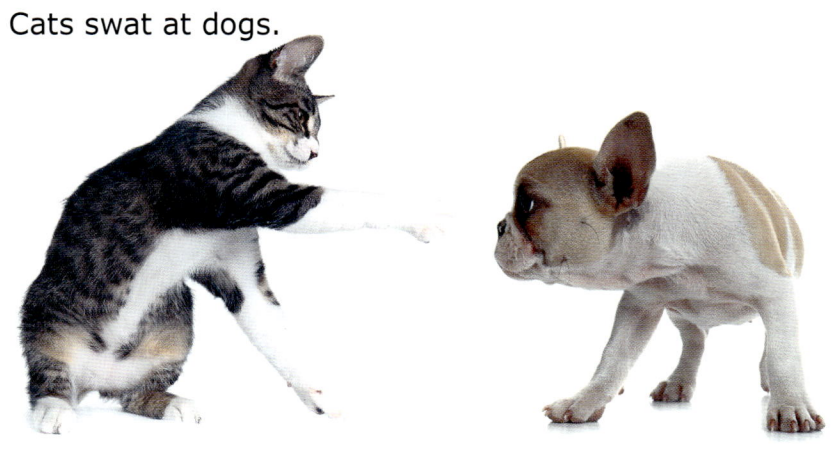

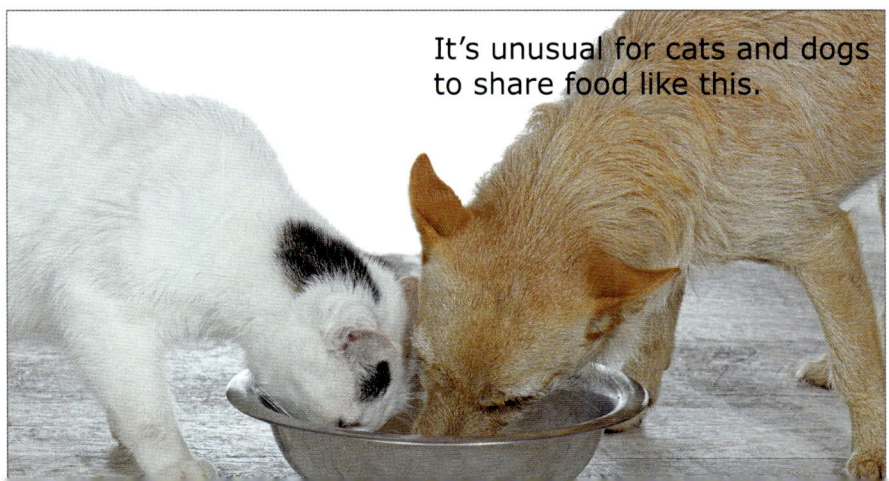

It's unusual for cats and dogs to share food like this.

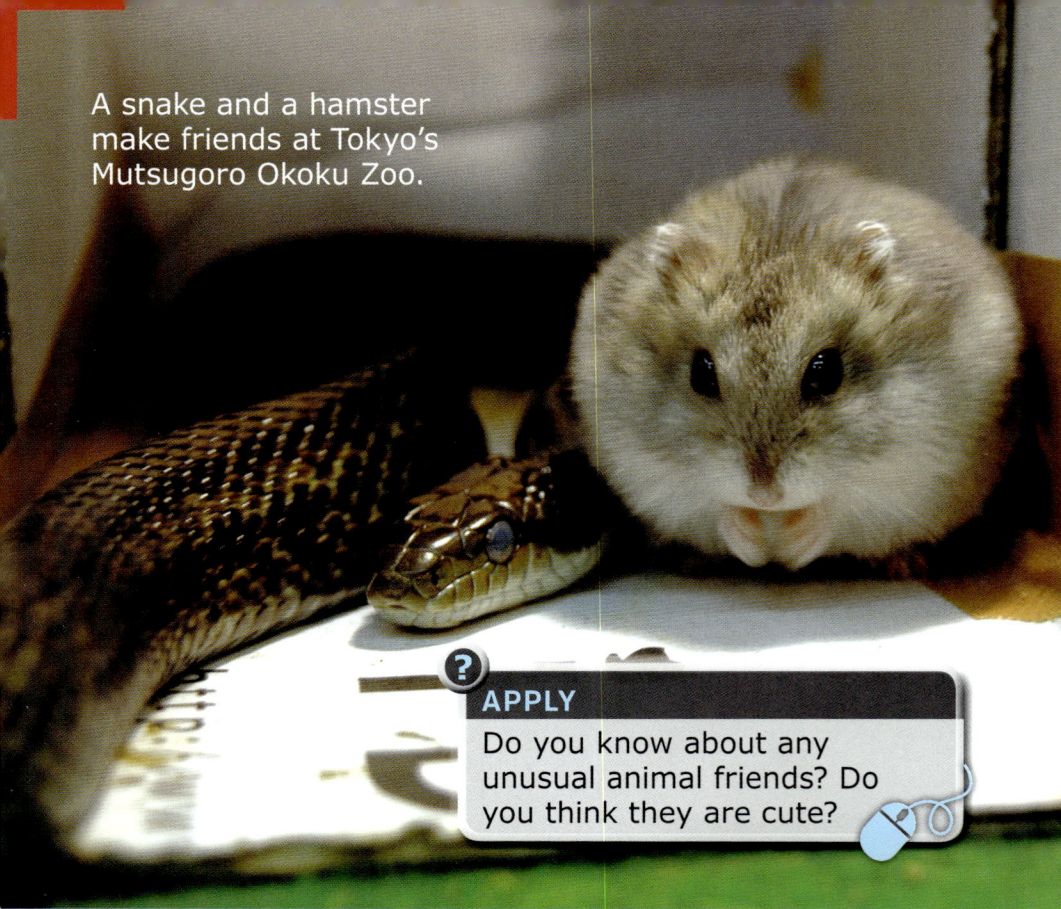

A snake and a hamster make friends at Tokyo's Mutsugoro Okoku Zoo.

APPLY

Do you know about any unusual animal friends? Do you think they are cute?

Animals can be dangerous. Different species often fight or even kill each other. So when we see two different species that are friends, we think it's cute. But can different species really be friends? Yes, they can.

On TV, in newspapers, and on the Internet, we see more and more stories of unusual animal friends. A few years ago, we even heard about a snake and a hamster who were friends at the Tokyo zoo.

Video Quest

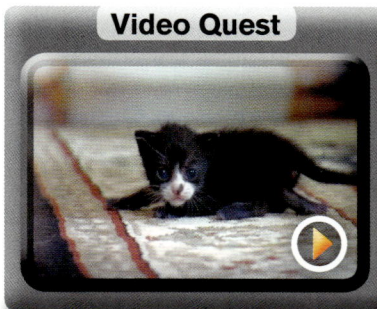

Are You My Mommy?

Watch the video. What is Oreo the kitten looking for?

Sometimes things go wrong in life. This is true for animals, too. Animals can lose a parent. Then the baby very often dies because there is no one to protect it. But sometimes an animal can find a new parent – a funny kind of adoption.[7]

In 2004, in Kenya, Africa, there was a baby hippo named Owen. Owen lost his family, so he went looking for a new mom. Mzee, a 130-year-old tortoise, took the job! A baby hippo with a tortoise mom – now, that's cute!

....

[7]**adoption:** making a baby or child part of your family

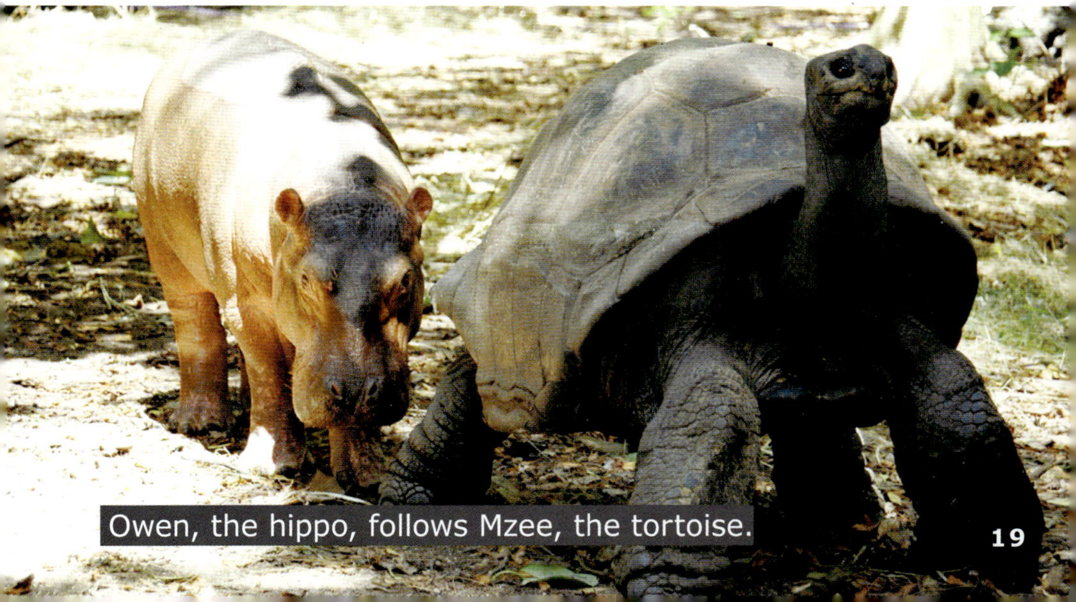

Owen, the hippo, follows Mzee, the tortoise.

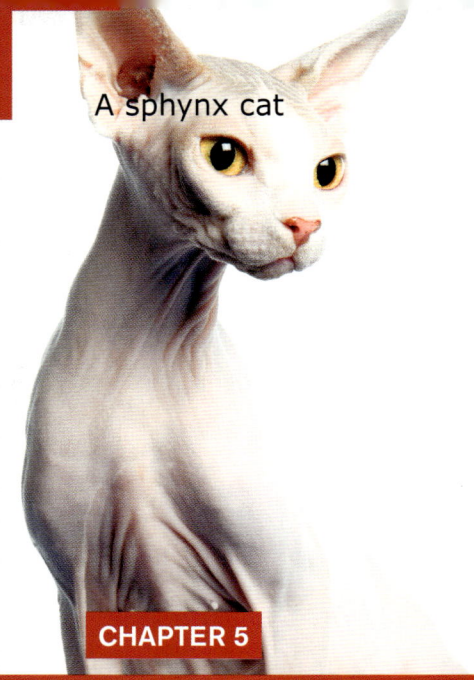
A sphynx cat

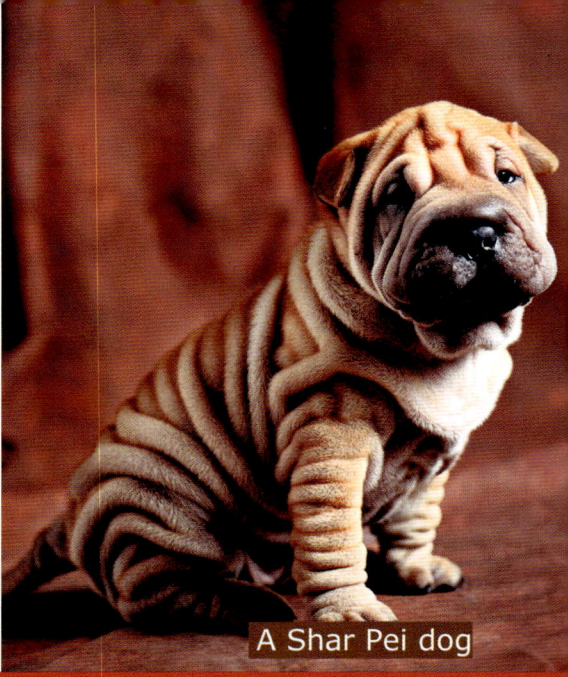
A Shar Pei dog

CHAPTER 5

What Do You Think?

BEAUTIFUL CAN BE CUTE. CAN UGLY ALSO BE CUTE?

For some people, very, very ugly is cute. For others very, very ugly is only ugly! Is it really possible that something is so ugly that it's cute?

There are cats with no hair and dogs with fat bodies and funny noses. Some people think they are very cute! Do you?

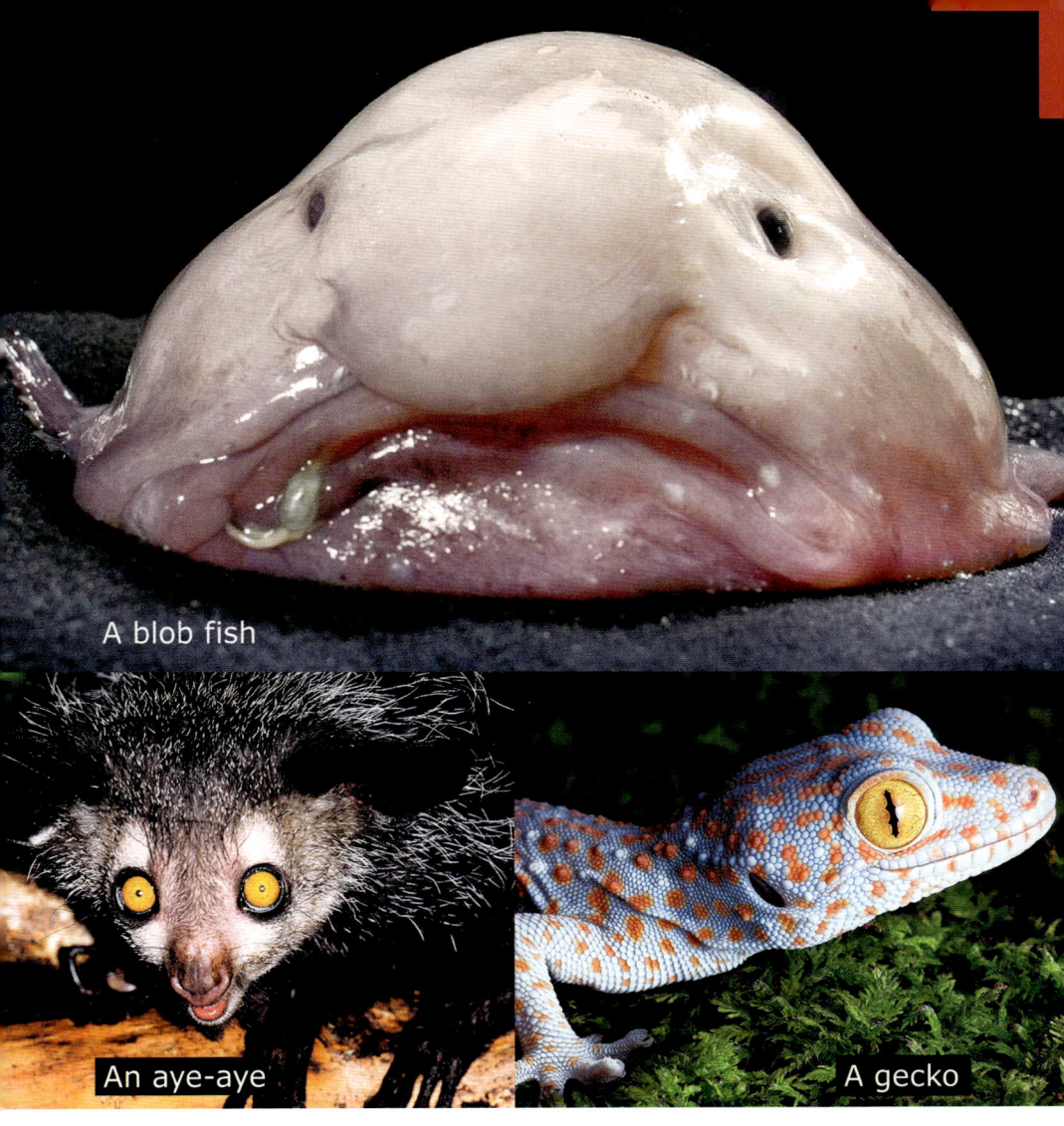

A blob fish

An aye-aye

A gecko

Look at the pictures. Are these animals cute or ugly?

So you can see that there are cute babies, kids, parents, and old people. There are even cute pictures.

What things in this book do you think are cute? Which picture really makes you say, "That's *so cute!*"?

After You Read

Read the sentences and choose Ⓐ (True) or Ⓑ (False).

1 Our brains tell us to protect cute people and animals.
- Ⓐ True
- Ⓑ False

2 Newborn puppies and kittens are helpless.
- Ⓐ True
- Ⓑ False

3 Animal babies never make mistakes.
- Ⓐ True
- Ⓑ False

4 Only human babies play.
- Ⓐ True
- Ⓑ False

5 We teach some animals to help people.
- Ⓐ True
- Ⓑ False

6 Hedgehogs have spikes.
- Ⓐ True
- Ⓑ False

7 Newborn birds don't need any help from their parents.
- Ⓐ True
- Ⓑ False

8 At a Tokyo zoo, a snake and a hippo are friends.
- Ⓐ True
- Ⓑ False

What Is Cute to Me?

Write down three things you think are cute. Why do you think they are cute?

What I find cute	Why it is cute
1.	
2.	
3.	

Complete the Sentences

Use the words in the box to complete the sentences.

brain	dangerous	helpless	laugh	older

1 When I see or hear something funny, I _____.

2 Watch out! These animals are _____ and can hurt you.

3 All humans, animals, and birds have a _____.

4 This baby can't do anything for himself. He's

_____ .

5 My brother was born three years before me. He's

_____ than I am.

Answer Key

Words to Know, page 4

1 ugly **2** Human babies **3** puppy **4** kids **5** kitten

Words to Know, page 5

1 brains **2** helpless **3** innocent **4** protect **5** mistakes **6** older

Apply, page 7

Answers will vary.

Video Quest, page 9

The babies are learning to play.

Evaluate, page 11

Answers will vary.

Video Quest, page 13

Teddy is learning to help people who can't see.

Understand, page 15

Puppies and kittens make mistakes like human babies do. They also behave badly at times.

Apply, page 18

Answers will vary.

Video Quest, page 19

Oreo is looking for a new family.

True or False?, page 22

1 A **2** A **3** B **4** B **5** A **6** A **7** B **8** B

What Is Cute to Me?, page 23

Answers will vary.

Complete the Sentences, page 23

1 laugh **2** dangerous **3** brain **4** helpless **5** older